# habit guide

## HOW TO BE HAPPY AND HEALTHY

Mike Kinnaird

*"We are what we repeatedly do.*
*Excellence, then, is not an act, but a habit."*

—Aristotle

# Contents

# ABOUT THE AUTHOR

One day at work something hit me like a ton of bricks. It was one of those pivotal moments we have in life. I was soldering— I was an electrical engineer and my head started swimming.

In only a couple of seconds I became disoriented, and right away was lost in a fog that was to last for 13 years.

I was scared. Suddenly I couldn't function, couldn't focus, couldn't do normal things like drive the car. I shut my whole life down. It was a knee-jerk reaction that was probably the wrong move but I didn't know what else to do. I lost everything and I mean… everything.

Those 13 years were pretty much torture. It was like having a permanent hang-over with flu as well. It was torture, hell—a living hell.

After spending years on the medical merry-go-round, with every specialist giving me a different diagnosis from inside his own "special" bag of tricks, I realized that medicine was not going to, and could not help me.

## LOOKING FOR ANSWERS

Enter phase two—the long and arduous search for the answers, because the health industry is a minefield of misinformation, debate, complexity, confusion and corruption.

Gradually, gradually through the frustration, the need for sanity and simplicity dawned. Finally, through a series of "ah-ha" moments, the truth dawned… the amazing, simple and glorious truth…

# "Nature"

We are a product of nature, our bodies are self-healing given the right conditions and if we look to nature, the answers are there. And they were.

## WHAT IS NATURAL?

Enter phase three—what *is* natural? The long search continued, and there's plenty of controversy here too. But search I did, and question and try, and stumble and fall. I left no stone unturned. By applying fierce logic and putting my conclusions into practice, I slowly started to feel better and better.

It's been a hell of a journey, and the madness of what I went through haunts me. The contrast between the two extreme states of my health fuels me with a passion you can only imagine—because all of my suffering was pointless, needless.

And all that torture was the result of being born into an unconscious world—a world unconscious of the importance of nature, the importance of lifestyle.

So… that's my story in as brief a way as I can make it, and the birth of *Habit Guide.* I just don't want anyone to suffer the misery that results from poor lifestyle—from decades of sub-optimal living, that chips away at health and happiness in the most insidious way.

As I wrote the book you're holding now, I always kept in mind, "What would you want Sam to know?" Samuel is my only son—only ten years old when *Habit Guide* was written. This proved to be an amazing writing mindset because I love him so much. I want only the best for Sam—that he's happy and healthy. I couldn't bear the thought of him suffering as I did.

Yet we're all someone's child, and we all want our children to be happy above all else.

I find it unbelievable now looking back, that in this day and age, so much suffering is still caused by ignorance of really simple truths about health and happiness.

So I've been incredibly passionate about bringing you this information—simple, clear guidance that puts the power of health and happiness in your hands. I hope with all my heart that you enjoy *Habit Guide*, that you put it to work, experience the amazing rewards, and never look back.

# FOREWORD

BY KATHRYN ELLIOTT

In my experience most people want to live well. They want wellbeing and vitality; the feeling that comes from being in the best of health. Moreover they understand there is a correlation between eating well, exercising and health.

Despite this people still struggle on a day-to-day basis, lacking the health and vitality they want and need to live well. While they may know the value of a good diet and lifestyle, the problem is how to do this.

Translating the desire to eat well and take care of yourself into a daily action plan can seem overwhelming. If you have to get kids to school, work a long day, take care of a family, maintain relationships—how do you find the time, resources and energy to look after your health?

It's in answering this question of how to live well that *Habit Guide* fits so perfectly. Mike has developed a brilliant resource that provides a road map to building good habits. A two week blitz of eating perfectly and exercising is not going to change your health long-term. Instead it's through building habits— daily and weekly practices—that you can change your health…

…which is the beauty of *Habit Guide*. It's a step-by-step guide to working out what you want, where you want to be, and how to get there.

*Kathryn Elliott is a nutritionist, herbalist and health educator from Sydney, Australia. Kathryn is an award-winning writer and contributes regular articles and recipe columns to a number of national publications.*

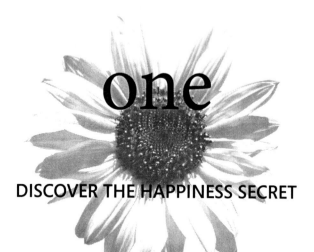

# one

## DISCOVER THE HAPPINESS SECRET

*"My life has no purpose, no direction, no aim, no meaning, and yet I'm happy. I can't figure it out. What am I doing right?"*

—Charles Schulz

Health and happiness creation is about just a few ideas pursued with dogged persistence.

And underlying the few ideas is just one principle that's so important, that without really harnessing it, all your attempts to be happy are doomed to failure.

This chapter is about the mindset of happiness… the mindset that leads to understanding just why that one principle is so important, and why it's overlooked—it's literally a secret.

It's a secret because it's tricky to understand and apply—so naturally, health professionals have tended to downplay it or miss it entirely.

I won't reveal the secret right away; because without the thought process that goes before it, you might not value it as much, or give it due care and attention—and it does deserve a lot of attention.

## THE CAUSES OF UNHAPPINESS

### WHERE ARE WE?

Nearly half of all deaths are caused by heart disease and cancer. Two thirds of Americans are overweight and one third of the adult population obese!

Very shocking—but what difference does it make how many, if *you* are sick and suffering? What does it matter how many, if *you* can't cope with life because you're depressed? And nobody ever thought it would be them to hear the words "I'm sorry to have to tell you; you have cancer."

But the statistics do tell a story; our modern lifestyles are causing pain and suffering on a massive scale.

Perhaps the saddest part of modern living is that our moods are flattened, and our joy for life snuffed out by poor lifestyles. Continuous stress and struggle becomes our accepted normality.

### WHERE DID IT ALL GO WRONG?

The very simple truth is that your genes expect a certain environment—the one that existed before the dawn of agriculture. That's only 500 generations ago or less, when we ate food directly from nature and had to work hard to get it.

In nature, genetics and the environment are exquisitely balanced because over time, the most well-adapted genes are passed on. So when our behavior or environment is out-of-sync with what our genes expect, we get sick and suffer.

The human body is incredibly adaptable. It's not that the environment needs to be so strictly defined. But what our bodies just cannot deal with is modern, processed and unnatural food, little exercise, and stress over decades. Although we can adapt well, there are limits that our bodies can cope with over a long time-frame.

The chronic diseases that are killing us, that make us sick, fat and depressed are even called "lifestyle diseases."

## A PILL FOR YOUR ILL?

If it's our lifestyles that are the root cause of chronic disease and unhappiness, is it reasonable to expect drugs or surgery to cure our ills?

It's very disempowering to believe that if you get sick, your doctor can bail you out, because it stops you taking responsibility for staying well now—being proactive.

You simply can't get health or happiness from a pill. Drugs are like using a sledge-hammer to crack your biochemical nut. Your biochemistry is incredibly complex and self-regulating given the right conditions. The true cure for any chronic disease is correction of the original cause—the reason it showed up in the first place.

Do you get a headache because your body lacks aspirin?

If someone's depressed, has their brain suddenly stopped making serotonin for no reason? Isn't it madness to treat depression with drugs that increase serotonin, if the cause is chronic lack of sleep, poor diet, overstimulation with caffeine, and a mindset that means they drive themselves to exhaustion?

Drugs often attempt to correct the symptom, the effect, and not the true cause. Antidepressants do nothing to affect the true causes, and so leave the poor person dependent on drugs to feel "normal." If the drug is stopped, the dysfunctional biochemistry is still there.

Isn't it madness to cut someone open and staple their stomach to stop them eating, when the person needs quality information, motivation, support, empowerment and permanent lifestyle shifts?

In many cases where drugs or surgery are used, there's a better way—a way that corrects the root cause of the problem.

Drugs exist because they sell, because we demand a quick fix. They sell because we buy into the pill-for-an-ill mindset and refuse or struggle or don't know how to change our behavior. What is demanded will be supplied—it always has and it always will.

## INFORMATION OVERLOAD

Once you've suffered enough pain from not living well, and once you've decided to put your health and happiness first, what do you do? You hunt for information… and pretty soon you're drowning in a sea of conflicting information about the best way to live.

Or perhaps with a "beginner's mind" you simply pick a book that looks good in the bookstore and throw yourself into the first program that appeals.

Either way isn't great. The seekers of the best lifestyle will rapidly become frustrated, because in every area of health, especially diet and exercise, there's very little agreement amongst "experts."

The one with beginner's mind is probably better off, but he or she is in a lottery. She may get lucky and pick up the right book, or she may not.

The advice you get from your bookstore is literally a lottery, which is quite a ridiculous state of affairs but nevertheless, that's where we are right now.

With exercise advice, it's not such a big deal but that's not true with nutrition. The advice you get is a very big deal indeed. Who's right you may wonder?

It's even more frustrating if you're trying to heal from disease. The hurdles to getting well are tough enough to leap, without the enormous task of trying to figure out which diet will work.

## WRONG FOCUS

When modern lifestyles squish our joy for life, it's natural for us to look for answers…

"It's my job that's making me unhappy, my partner, I have too much to do, I can't relax. I need a new car, a new career, a new house. I need to be appreciated, I need to be successful…" ad infinitum.

It's not that any of these things don't matter. Of course they do. But your life is primarily a reflection of your *inner state*.

To be happy, go after happiness *directly!*

It's about the right focus and the right priorities. Change your inner state first, then, as if by magic, your outer life will fall in line with the new you.

I got chatting to a guy on my walkabout one day… He'd been to the shops to buy his favorite rump steak—he eats red meat twice a day, and then he'd called in at the bar for his daily 3 pints of beer.

He told me he had high blood pressure, gout and arthritis, for which he took a total of 8 pills a day. After a lot of talking, it turned out the thing he wanted most is… health!

Let's assume, on a scale of 1 to 10, his feel-good-factor is wavering between 2 and 5 and averages about 3.5. In other words, like most people, he doesn't feel great. He struggles with energy and doesn't think so clearly, and so he's not coping so well with just about everything. This is really common, life feeling like a drudge.

And then comes beer time, or steak time… or if he's really lucky, steak and beer time! The pleasure is pushing his feel-good-factor up to 6 or 7 all of a sudden. He feels good again.

But let's say he decides to be healthier, and starts denying himself the things that are bad for his health. Now comes the detox and instead of averaging a 3.5 on the feel-good scale, he's dropping to 2 or even 1. He feels worse, and now doesn't even get the little pleasures in life, the very things that to him make life worth living.

This scenario is why sustained efforts to change are quite rare, and folks tend to mentally "settle" with "I'll do whatever and let the chips fall where they may."

That's a shame, that's sad, because what we want is to feel the best we can. The low vitality pleasure seekers are doing the best they can to achieve the best feelings, but it's a long way from what's possible.

This is settling for a poor existence, compared to what's possible when you understand the big picture—that declining vitality is forcing you to look to pleasure as your only way to feel good. And those little pleasures last for such a short time, before you're back to 3.5.

We want to feel good, that's *all* we want.

A better way is to raise vitality to a 7 or 8 or even higher... a natural high.

When your vitality is high, you stop pleasure seeking as a way to feel good, because you already feel good.

So the norm is declining vitality, peaked by moments of pleasure, which can become psychological or physical addictions. That's not living. And most of the pleasures we live for cause vitality to drop over the long term.

So in a few years, a 3.5 is going to be more like 2.5. And as our vitality begins to bottom out, the urge to self-medicate our bad feelings with our usual fix becomes irresistible—we can end up in a vicious circle of self-destruction.

I want you to experience a 10 on the feel-good scale. 3.5 sucks! Don't settle... aim for a natural high, the natural feel good that is yours for the taking. Once you're done with the change part, once you've healed, doing the things that keep you naturally high do not feel like denial. It's actually a joy to do the things that will keep you bouncing along.

## THE CAUSES OF HAPPINESS

KNOWING WHAT

The causes of happiness are health and peace of mind. Think about how happy children are... they have high energy, no worries, no hang-ups, and live in the present moment—the causes of happiness.

This could be everyone's natural state, but decades of not living well and too much stress eats into our vitality—the vitality and peace of mind that children naturally have.

But your body is very forgiving. It can heal and given the right conditions; go back to a state of health and vitality. And by giving ourselves a serious *reality* check, we can re-connect to the present moment, and gain the peace of mind that brings spontaneity, laughter and joy.

There are six lifestyle elements that you need to be aware of every day, to make sure that these causes of happiness are consistently there. The first four are about creating health and the last two are about creating peace of mind…

1. Eat and drink the right stuff

2. Be free from drugs

3. Exercise outdoors

4. Sleep well

5. Get organized

6. Live in the moment

## KNOWING HOW

Ideally, we would have been born into a world where the causes of happiness were widely understood, embedded into our culture, and we simply learned the wisdom from an early age.

But it's not so easy for you and me, because we need to *undo* all the misinformation and behaviors that take us away from joy and happiness.

All this undoing falls into the realm of *how*—how to change, how to finally end up with all the causes of happiness in place every day for life.

So… how do we get from here to there? How do we see the big picture, see the finish line, manage detox, manage change and so-on?

Well, change is truly the tricky part. Once you've arrived at high vitality, living that way is *easy*. Then it's just as easy to stay feeling good, as it was to stay feeling bad.

Coming from the lowest vitality and quality of life you can imagine, my need to change was immense. And I stumbled into all the problems that I now see everyone else stumbling into.

The way from here to there takes a little explaining, so I've compiled "the way" into the rest of the book. It will show you how to navigate the pitfalls and obstacles to a happy life, full of vitality, and hit your natural high.

## HAVING THE RIGHT MINDSET

Apart from the big ones like "nature" and the "two causes of happiness," there's a couple of other crucial mindset distinctions you need…

### Everything affects everything else

This is essentially the opposite of the pill-for-an-ill mindset. The truth is that everything affects everything else. It's easy to see how a few bad nights' sleep can affect every interaction, relationship and decision. But these connections run very deep indeed. Whether or not you get cancer in twenty years depends on what's on your fork today.

Everything affects every other thing.

That's why we need a whole lifestyle, multi-pronged strategy. It's only when your whole lifestyle is right, that you can experience the wonderful feelings of permanent energy and health.

**Checking health boxes is your number one priority**

Because we are now outside the controls of nature, we must consciously *choose* to check health boxes, every day. All our instincts work in a natural environment, they don't work at all well in modern life.

For example, our fight or flight response kicks in at the most inappropriate times—like being stuck in traffic. Or we crave high-fat, high-sugar combination foods like pizza and ice-cream that drive our taste buds wild with excitement. These types of food never existed until recently.

It's so easy to get distracted with a million things to do, but decide for yourself—what's really important?

What you decide is important to you, is very important. If you know and understand with incredible clarity, that without checking health boxes every single day, you won't be happy, then you make that important in your mind. You have the right attitude—"This comes first, it's more important than any other thing," because health is fundamental. It's the foundational state of a happy life.

When you have amazing energy and clarity, your life will automatically go in wonderful new directions that you can't even imagine right now!

That's why health is number one.

Happiness is built on a consistent lifestyle. Exercise is not the answer... daily exercise is the answer. Good food is not the answer... good food every day is the answer. No single factor is the answer except the secret.

Happiness is about lots of things because everything affects everything else.

Now we have clear mental distinctions—a new mindset and motivation to check health boxes every day.

So what's the one principle that underlies all these things? What's the one crucial factor you must harness? (Drum roll)...

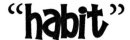

You probably guessed, reading a book called *Habit Guide!*

OK, it's not a glamorous word, but it's our *habits* that drive our thoughts and actions. We couldn't walk, talk, or tie our shoe laces without habits, and the habit connections run very deep.

Good habits make the conditions for happiness effortless and that's the key. It's consistency; it's doing all the good things consistently. And to do that you need habit power, because habit is the power that effortlessly repeats.

Habit doesn't care whether your behavior is good or bad, it repeats anyway. So we get incredibly clear and we harness habit power—break bad habits, and put new ones in place that create happiness and joy for life.

*"HABIT IS THE DEEPEST LAW OF HUMAN NATURE."*

—Thomas Carlyle

Habit is the deepest law! When we do something without thinking about it, we say it's *second nature*.

That's a powerful truth to ponder. Once you know something, you start to see it everywhere. And now you know that it's your habits that build health and happiness, you'll start to notice it too.

But it's not enough to know it; you need to put the power of habit to work in your life.

And this is the book that will empower you to do just that. It will show you precisely what you need to do every day and how to do it, to actually *be* happy! It will give you the tools you need to break stubborn bad habits and create healthy new ones—the powerful causes of health and happiness.

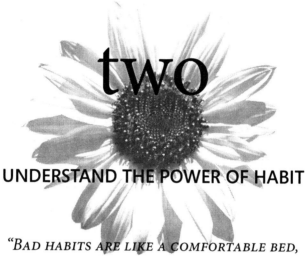

# two

## UNDERSTAND THE POWER OF HABIT

*"BAD HABITS ARE LIKE A COMFORTABLE BED,*
*EASY TO GET INTO, BUT HARD TO GET OUT OF."*

—Proverb

People leading happy and healthy lives aren't constantly resisting temptation. Their lifestyle is effortless.

It doesn't mean they're stronger willed than you are. Happy and healthy people are often unwittingly using the power of habit to generate the outcome of health, just as those in bad habits are using the power of habit to create the outcome of poor health.

It's change that we find so difficult—undoing years of bad habits and creating that effortless healthy lifestyle, with all the benefits that come with it.

I love this analogy of self-destructive habits:

*"A FLY IN A PITCHER PLANT IS,*
*AT THE BEGINNING EATING THE PLANT.*
*AT SOME IMPERCEPTIBLE POINT,*
*THE PLANT IS EATING THE FLY"*

In the beginning we have choice, but gradually over the years, our habits begin to dominate our behavior more and more and we become slaves to them—set in our *ways*.

## HABITS ARE SUBTLE AND POWERFUL

Look at your life for a second. How much of what you do is routine or habit—stuff that you do every day, without even thinking? Even the way we think is largely habit.

Our thoughts, like our behavior, consist mainly of reactions that have been previously conditioned. This is a good thing, we need it, and it's an essential aspect of learning. If we didn't have this part to ourselves we wouldn't be able to function in life at all.

Every day we act out our learned behavior. The key to changing your life is to change what you do and think—your routines and habits.

Think about the last time you parked your car in a public place. Chances are you hunted for "your" spot, where you always park. Or how about which shops you go in? Which websites you look at? What you have for your meals? Who you speak to? What you do in your spare time? They're all pretty much the same most of the time.

Habit comforts us, and it makes it easier to navigate life. We like what we know—we love being in our comfort zones and it feels bad when we aren't... when there is no "programming," no mental map as to what's going on.

One time at the gym, workmen were working on the path so my usual route out of the front door was blocked. For two weeks I still turned to go my normal way, even though I knew the path was being fixed. By the time I was "reprogrammed," they'd finished the work and it took me another two weeks to reprogram myself back again! Such is the power of habit.

But habits are also the stumbling block of attempts to change our lives. These subtle but powerful forces dominate everything we do. Often, we know what we want but we don't quite know how to get it.

The fact is that we're constantly and consistently responding to external and internal triggers that cause us to behave in certain ways. There are many factors involved in this conditioning, and in the main they serve us well.

It's only when our conditioning has unpleasant consequences, or when we keep trying to change and fail, that we realize that a lot of the time, we don't have choice or freedom.

## A GROOVY MIND

Our conditioning in many ways defines who we are. In our unique upbringing we are constantly and repeatedly "molded" by our parents and peers to have certain values and learn certain things.

We think that the values we hold so dear are part of "us." It's true, we can and do think for ourselves but many of our values represent conditioning, especially childhood conditioning. But what's this got to do with habits?

Well, imagine… you're born and your mind is like a smooth, blank, vinyl record. The only track on there is a little track called "instinct." The rest of the vinyl starts to get written on as you grow—language skills, walking, eating and later—ideas, concepts, values and experience.

Our mind differs from the vinyl though, its grooves are multi-dimensional and can interlink with each other. Also, the mind can automatically play along many grooves at once as well as recording at the same time, without any effort from us—amazing!

All of life's experience is written in our mind grooves and each groove has its own volume, or depth. The depth depends on two things. Firstly, the number of times you have the experience and secondly, the intensity of the experience.

Compulsive behavior is caused by very deep grooves, often initially caused by a traumatic event. Destructive habits are caused by very deep grooves, caused by repetition.

Our unconscious mind runs along these grooves and the deeper they are, the harder it is for us to consciously override or change the programming.

When we encounter a trigger in our lives, we go into an automatic unconscious groove of learned behavior.

So, repetition and intensity are the two main factors that deepen those mental grooves. Our physical habits, the things we do, reflect our mental habits. If our lives have lots of deep grooves (routines and habits) that don't support what we want to achieve, we say we're "in a rut."

## SKILLS ARE JUST COMPLEX HABITS

Imagine a dancer. A dancer trains for years, perfecting her "grooves" by consciously programming the vinyl of the mind to run along precisely the right grooves. On performance night, she triggers the start and the rest is automatic. She doesn't consciously do anything.

Same thing when you learned to drive, speak, do martial arts, play the guitar or any skill whatsoever. You put in conscious effort to make it eventually automatic. The more automatic and the more complex, the more we have mastered the skill.

We even refer to this in language when we say "It's like riding a bike," to mean once learned, you never forget. You can do it easily, only when you can finally stop consciously thinking about it.

So, by mastering the subtle force of habit, you can tap into an incredibly powerful way to make sure you do the things you need to do every day, to always feel good—auto health and happiness.

# three

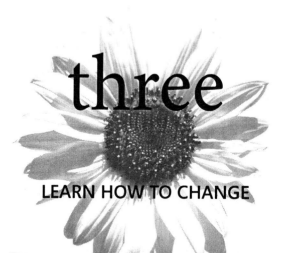

## LEARN HOW TO CHANGE

*"HABIT IS EITHER THE BEST OF SERVANTS,*
*OR THE WORST OF MASTERS."*

—Nathaniel Emmons

Without the right information, successful change is rare because old habits die hard. Habits are very subtle and powerful—quite a combination! To be successful, you need to know how to get habit power working for you.

First we'll look at the big picture and then the detail…

### THE BIG PICTURE OF CHANGE

If you can master two things, you can master "how to" create health and peace of mind—the conditions for happiness. These two things are…

1. How to DO something (develop good habits)

2. How to NOT DO something (break bad habits)

Simply put, to get yourself to do something, keep your mind *on it*. To not do something, keep your mind *off it*. So, all the tools for both 1 and 2 have the aim of either keeping your attention on something or off it.

Understanding the power of attention is possibly the most important information you could ever learn. What we pay attention to grows, what we remove attention from, dies away. Attention is the volume control for thoughts.

This knowledge has far reaching consequences for everything in your life...

## You have the power of choice, and you choose with your attention

## DEVELOP GOOD HABITS

Your brain is wired for association and habit so developing good habits is much easier than breaking bad ones. It's all about deciding your next step, and keeping your mind on it when it's time to do it.

Before you begin, you need to set up **a pact.**

This is a clear and calm decision to follow through with your next step. This step should not be too far outside your comfort zone—the weeks go by quickly and you end up getting nowhere by false-starting.

We want wins and getting wins will increase your self-belief. Make each week count and make consistent, sure-footed steps towards your finish line—the final outcome you choose.

Your pact should be very simple with the absolute minimum of ifs, buts and maybes.

These three tips will really help establish your new good habit:

1. **Link it.** If possible, link your new habit to another activity you already do. If you want to start exercising then link it to say, getting home from work or some other event or action. This way you'll never forget, and you'll build powerful associations that make doing the good thing easy.

2. **Keep your mind on it.** Keep thinking about doing it until it resolves into action—until you actually get up and do it.

3. **Do it a little bit.** Always follow through with the new habit, even if you just do it a little bit. This way you keep the habit going and that's the important thing.

We are building habits for life—good habits that remind and urge you to do good things. That's going to mean you stay happy, healthy and feeling good!

## BREAK BAD HABITS

Before reading on, don't think of a pink elephant for 30 seconds.

You can't tell your mind not to think about something. The way to keep your mind off something, is to think about *something else.*

So, to break your bad habits you need to understand "attention flow." This is your moment-to-moment attention when you get an urge to do bad things.

Before you begin, you need to set up **a pact.**

This is a clear and calm decision to follow through with your next step, to choose long-term vitality over the quick fix. This step should not be too far outside your comfort zone—the weeks go by quickly and you end up getting nowhere by false-starting.

We want wins and getting wins will increase your self-belief. Make each week count and make consistent, sure-footed steps towards your finish line. Knowing your finish line and your next step will allow you to drop *the problem*—all the worry and analysis that gives attention to the very thing you're trying to stop.

Your pact should be very simple with the absolute minimum of ifs, buts and maybes.

Once you have a pact, **ignore** any thought or feeling that goes against it. Have a "don't care" attitude towards the arising thoughts or feelings. See them as just the old pattern and bring your full attention back to what you were doing—pay no attention to your pink elephant.

Ride out any backlash, whether it's physical (tiredness), mental (I'll start tomorrow), emotional (tantrum) or a combination—this feeling will pass.

Simply persist, no matter what the frequency or intensity of arising thoughts or urges.

This simple method gives you the power to reprogram or eliminate all habits—not just physical habits but thought habits too. You can use it to choose behavior, alter the way you react to emotions and get rid of unwanted thoughts.

As you get into the habit of "listening" to your thoughts—more on that in the Live in the Moment chapter, you'll find it easier and easier to ignore unwanted thoughts and choose the focus of your attention.

# four

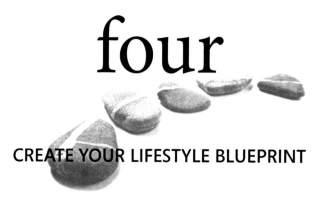

## CREATE YOUR LIFESTYLE BLUEPRINT

*"It takes a lot of aspirin to feel good*
*if you're sitting on a tack."*

—Tack Law, Sydney MacDonald Baker, M.D.

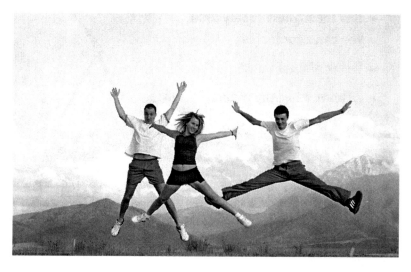

The *Habit Guide* lifestyle blueprint is a model lifestyle you can use to create your own. As you read through the lifestyle chapters, have a think about how you're going to apply each one to your life. It will help a lot when it comes to taking action later on.

Although the list of human needs is very long, the lifestyle blueprint is just the things that need your conscious attention every day. It's those needs that without attention will not be met consistently, and so you'll suffer as a result—lack of energy, depression, disease and so-on.

Your needs like fun, nurture, community, passion, and love will be met automatically *because* of your vitality, energy and happiness. Everything affects everything else.

## EAT AND DRINK THE RIGHT STUFF

- Eat whole, natural foods. 3 meals and 2 snacks.

- Follow the *Habit Guide* diet.

- Buy the highest quality food you can afford.

- Drink filtered water.

- Achieve a healthy weight.

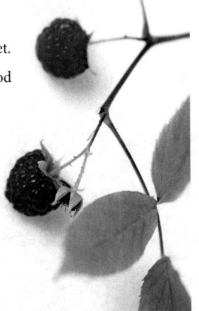

- Talk to your doctor about the conditions needed to reduce your medication.

- Beware common drugs—caffeine, nicotine, alcohol and so-on.

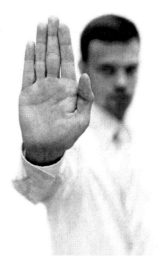

## EXERCISE

- Above all, find something you enjoy.

- Aerobic exercise or sports *outdoors,* 30 minutes, Monday to Friday.

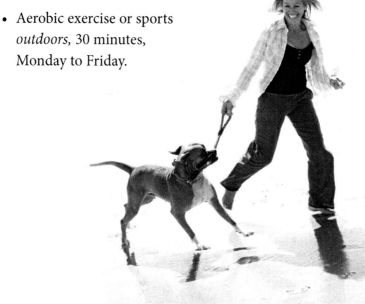

- Get into a regular routine. Shift by no more than 1 hour if possible at the weekend.

- Practice full-body relaxation before sleep.

- Use black-out curtains and a dawn simulation lamp.

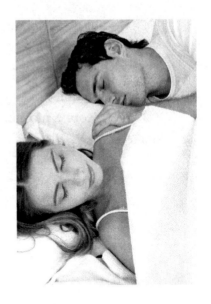

## GET ORGANIZED

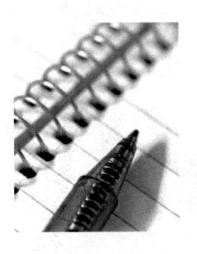

- Free your mind from worry by systemizing.

- Follow our simple system for keeping track of your projects and obligations.

- If it isn't being used or isn't beautiful, get rid of it! What you own ends up owning you.

- Create a harmonious, simple and beautiful place to be. Do you feel good in your surroundings?

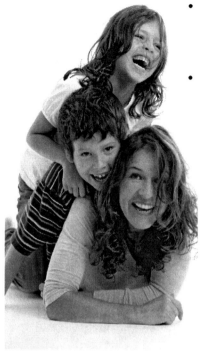

- Drop the mind-chatter and you're there—or rather *here, now.*

- Set a relaxed pace.

# five

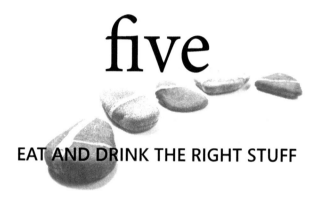

## EAT AND DRINK THE RIGHT STUFF

*"Let food be thy medicine
and medicine be thy food."*

—Hippocrates

THE HABIT GUIDE DIET

What's on your fork today contributes to your health and happiness in a week, a year, ten years, fifty years—your health "outcomes."

And we like what we know. If you get onto a healthy eating plan, you'll come to love it, cravings will drop away and you'll get happier and happier.

What you eat is a huge part of the happiness equation.

The truth is that your body has a lot of needs when it comes to nutrition. It's a long list that science has identified—the components of food like fiber, vitamins, minerals, phytonutrients, essential fats and so-on.

There's another long list of things we eat a lot of that we really shouldn't eat—too much saturated fat, sugar, excess salt, too much overall fat, trans fats, refined carbohydrates, high GI food, processed foods, additives and so-on.

The big reason we eat a lot of the bad list is that it drives our taste buds wild, but your instincts only work with natural foods, not with pizza, ice-cream or chocolate.

So, how can we make sure we get all our needs every single day? How can we avoid all that stuff that's bad for us, and enjoy the food that's good for our bodies and not just our taste buds?

The only sane answer is *structure*.

The main point is to develop a simple meal structure, that you repeat every day but with different foods. That way, you can be confident of getting your good nutrition for the days, months, and years ahead.

The benefits of simple changes—like having a daily salad, getting vegetables with your evening meal, plus adding a fruit starter to every meal, stack up when you repeat them every day.

Of course, daily events can sometimes throw you off course and you can't always follow your plan. No worries—it's what you do most of the time that matters.

So, the daily diet plan on the next page is exactly what to eat and a simple way to get all those things you need, and avoid those things you'd be better off not eating...

# DAILY DIET PLAN

**Smoothie**

1 or 2 bananas, apples or pears

1 scoop protein powder e.g. soy, hemp, pea, whey, egg. Vary the type used

Fresh or frozen berries or other fruit

Option: 1 or 2 sticks celery or lettuce

Milk substitute e.g. soy, rice

*Directions:* Blend

Handful of nuts or seeds

1 multivitamin + minerals, 2 fish oil capsules

**Starter** 1 or 2 pieces fruit

**Main course salad**

Salad greens e.g. lettuce, watercress, spinach, arugula

Salad vegetables e.g. cucumber, tomato, bell pepper

Lean protein e.g. chicken breast, pork, fish, tofu, egg, beans, lentils

Gluten-free whole grains e.g. quinoa, rice, millet

High quality salad dressing

DINNER

**Starter** 1 or 2 pieces fruit

**Main course**

Lean protein e.g. chicken breast, fish, meat etc.

2 fresh or frozen steamed/roasted vegetables

New potatoes, sweet potatoes, yams or squashes

Sauce *or* occasionally butter or olive oil

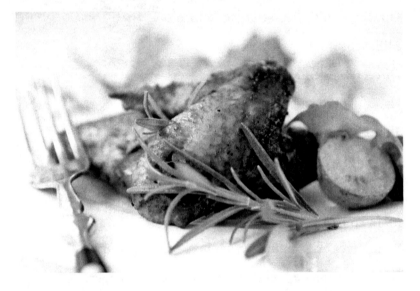

**Snacks** Fruit + yogurt *or* raw vegetable crudités + dip e.g. hummus, guacamole, salsa *or* a handful of nuts

Color diet sheets for you to print out and stick on your fridge are available at www.habitguide.com/diet-sheets

MEAL TIMING

Ideally, time your meals so you're not going longer than four hours without a feed. So a typical day might be:

| 8.00am | Breakfast |
|--------|-----------|
| 12.00pm | Lunch |
| 4.00pm | Snack |
| 6.00pm | Dinner |
| 10.00pm | Snack |

## TAKING STOCK

Keep a stock list—amounts of the different types of food you need to keep in the house. Stock levels will vary depending on the size of your family. It's a balancing act that when you get right, will mean there's always enough to put a quick meal together, but you're not throwing gone-off food away.

Keep tweaking your list until you get that balance just right. Then it's a simple matter of figuring out what you need to buy to get back to "full stock" when it's time to go grocery shopping.

## A FEW NOTES ON THE DIET

- This is a diet that's high in fruits and vegetables. It's a big step back to eating natural human foods and has the feel good, convenience and taste factors that will make it work in your real life.

- Grains and dairy are not natural foods for humans so it's a low grain, gluten-free diet, having probably a third or less of the grains of a typical Western diet. Dairy use is limited to yogurt as a snack option and the occasional bit of butter with dinner.

- Unnatural foods have the potential to cause real upset in your body. They contain things that your body could have real problems dealing with and they can cause a cascade of symptoms that then cause other problems. In the end, the dots can be very difficult to connect— it can be really hard to identify the true cause of our problems. If you have existing unresolved and long-term health issues, I recommend eliminating grains and dairy altogether.

- Check with your doctor before taking fish oil if you are taking blood thinning medication.

- Have fish twice per week—at least one being oily fish (salmon, mackerel, sardines, tuna, trout) or if you're vegetarian: a teaspoon of flax seed oil every day. This is important for omega-3 fatty-acids.

- Reduce or eliminate stimulants of all kinds (such as tea and coffee) as these can disturb your natural appetite and instincts, and contribute to blood sugar disorders.

- Take the time to really enjoy your food. Eat slowly and chew your food properly.

- If you're vegetarian you can still follow the *Habit Guide* diet plan using vegetarian sources of protein instead of fish/meat.

- If you want grains with dinner, then have your starchy vegetables with lunch.

- Leftover steamed vegetables for dinner can be kept in the fridge overnight and added to your lunch-time salad the next day.

- If you need to lose weight, follow the weight loss plan below.

- Vitamin D is low on this diet as with any natural diet. Vitamin D is the sunshine vitamin so you'll want to be getting outdoors. Your multivitamin will provide 100% RDA of vitamin D as a safety measure.

If you follow the *Habit Guide* diet, you'll automatically check all the nutrition boxes and avoid the harmful stuff.

## ACHIEVE A HEALTHY WEIGHT

This is the simplest and most effective weight loss plan you'll ever find! It's effective because by getting into good habits you can hit your target weight easily. *And* you'll have the habits installed that not only keep you slim, but happy and healthy for life.

To lose weight, all we need to do is take the powerful elements of the *Habit Guide* diet and eat a little bit less of it. It's this extreme clarity of what to do each day, that will mean steady and sustained weight loss without the yo-yoing.

It is *structure* that will give you the clarity and confidence of knowing exactly what you're doing, and the result it's having. So let's get on with it!

WEIGHT LOSS PLAN

Below are 1750, 1500 and 1250 calorie versions of the *Habit Guide* diet. Simply pick the one that's right for you and get started!

| | | |
|---|---|---|
| **Men** | More than 225lbs | 1750 |
| | Less than 225lbs | 1500 |
| **Women** | More than 200lbs | 1500 |
| | Less than 200lbs | 1250 |

# 1750 PLAN

BREAKFAST SMOOTHIE ~ 300
½ oz protein powder (50)
½ pc fruit—banana, apple, pear (40)
4½ oz fresh or frozen berries (40)
6 oz milk substitute (85)
½ oz nuts or seeds (85)
1 multivitamin, 2 fish oil capsules

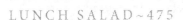

LUNCH SALAD ~ 475
Starter: 2 pieces medium fruit (160)
1-1½ oz salad greens (5)
4 oz salad vegetables—cucumber, tomato, bell pepper etc. (20)
3 oz lean protein—chicken, fish, tofu, egg whites etc. (140)
3 oz cooked quinoa, rice or millet (100)
½ oz high quality salad dressing (50)

SNACK 1 ~ 100: ½ pc fruit + 60 cals yogurt or vegetable
crudités + 1½ oz hummus or guacamole

DINNER ~ 475
Starter: 1 pc fruit (80)
3 oz lean protein—chicken breast, fish, meat etc. (140)
4 oz fresh or frozen steamed/roasted vegetables (80)
4 oz cooked new potatoes or sweet potatoes (110)
Sauce *or* 2 tsp butter *or* 2 tsp olive oil (65)

*Or* repeat lunch *or* 475 cals of something else!

SNACK 2 ~ 100: ½ pc fruit + 60 cals yogurt *or* vegetable
crudités + 1½ oz hummus or guacamole

EXTRAS ~ 300: Drinks, chocolate, alcohol etc.

# 1500 PLAN

BREAKFAST SMOOTHIE~300
½ oz protein powder (50)
½ pc fruit—banana, apple, pear (40)
4½ oz fresh or frozen berries (40)
6 oz milk substitute (85)
½ oz nuts or seeds (85)
1 multivitamin, 2 fish oil capsules

LUNCH SALAD~400
Starter: 1 piece medium fruit (80)
1-1½ oz salad greens (5)
4 oz salad vegetables—cucumber, tomato, bell pepper etc. (20)
3 oz lean protein—chicken, fish, tofu, egg whites etc. (140)
3 oz cooked quinoa, rice or millet (100)
½ oz high quality salad dressing (50)

SNACK 1~100: ½ pc fruit + 60 cals yogurt or vegetable
crudités + 1½ oz hummus or guacamole

DINNER~400
Starter: 1 pc fruit (80)
3 oz lean protein—chicken breast, fish, meat etc. (140)
3 oz fresh or frozen steamed/roasted vegetables (60)
2 oz cooked new potatoes or sweet potatoes (55)
Sauce *or* 2 tsp butter *or* 2 tsp olive oil (65)

*Or* repeat lunch *or* 400 cals of something else!

SNACK 2~100: ½ pc fruit + 60 cals yogurt *or* vegetable
crudités + 1½ oz hummus or guacamole

EXTRAS~200: Drinks, chocolate, alcohol etc.

# 1250 PLAN

½ oz protein powder (50)
½ pc fruit—banana, apple, pear (40)
3½ oz fresh or frozen berries (30)
6 oz milk substitute (85)

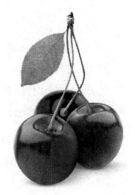

¼ oz nuts or seeds (45)
1 multivitamin, 2 fish oil capsules

LUNCH SALAD~300
Starter: ½ piece medium fruit (40)
1-1½ oz salad greens (5)
4 oz salad vegetables—cucumber, tomato, bell pepper etc. (20)
2½ oz lean protein—chicken, fish, tofu, egg whites etc. (115)
2 oz cooked quinoa, rice or millet (70)
½ oz high quality salad dressing (50)

SNACK 1~100: ½ pc fruit + 60 cals yogurt or vegetable crudités + 1½ oz hummus or guacamole

DINNER~300
Starter: ½ pc fruit (40)
2½ oz lean protein—chicken breast, fish, meat etc. (115)
2 oz fresh or frozen steamed/roasted vegetables (40)
2 oz cooked new potatoes or sweet potatoes (55)
Sauce *or* 1½ tsp butter *or* 1½ tsp olive oil (50)

*Or* repeat lunch *or* 300 cals of something else!

SNACK 2~100: ½ pc fruit + 60 cals yogurt *or* vegetable crudités + 1½ oz hummus or guacamole

EXTRAS~200: Drinks, chocolate, alcohol etc.

With the *Habit Guide* diet you can make a meal with whatever is in the fridge and fruit bowl. It's tasty food fast that hits your calorie target for that meal, with no thinking or stressing. That's what's going to get the job done.

The calorie figures on each plan are there in case you want to swap out any ingredients, or even the whole meal. The plans are templates, not rigid diets. It's what you do if nothing else comes up—it's your "default" day.

So, you don't need to get each separate food item to match the calories. The calories for each food item are averaged out so you only need to get a variety of fruits, vegetables, and so-on, over the course of your week—and then get the portion sizes right.

It's important to stick to the meal timings so if you're out and about, or haven't had time to prep the salad, eat whatever you can that matches the calorie target for that meal. Obviously make the healthiest choice you can, but if all you can find is potato chips, then eat those. Don't skip meals!

It's usually only the evening meal that could cause problems. With such a healthy breakfast and lunch, you can still fit in with the family when dieting. If your family wants pizza and you want to join them, then look on the packaging, and it's easy enough to figure out how much you can have and still stay on track.

Another very easy option is to make up two portions of the salad meal, and have half for lunch and half for dinner. Food is nutrition remember—quality fuel for your body. We can take the stress out of being healthy and dieting, by dropping the idea that every meal has to be Michelin starred.

If your partner wants to join in with you, then it's very easy. If one of you is doing the 1250 plan and the other the 1750, it's simply a case of weighing out the different portion sizes for each of you. You both get to go at your own speed without having to cook up different food.

## EASY DOES IT

Whichever of the 3 plans is right for you, there's no need to dive straight in. Almost everyone can start with the 1750 plan and start to lose weight. Give yourself time to ease into these new habits—to get used to making the new meals, stocking up, and getting your family used to what's happening. Also, it gives your body a chance to adapt—hormones and enzyme reactions don't change overnight.

By easing your way into this, you'll gain confidence as you go, and get used to what it feels like to be at the 1750 level. When you see how easy it is, you'll be spurred on to move to the 1500 and then 1250, if that's the plan for you.

## SAUCY

The plans allow for 65 or 50 calories of sauce, butter, or olive oil to put on the dinner meal. There's no need to have those horrible low-fat sauces full of chemicals just because you're on a weight loss plan! Urgh! The plans allow for plenty of flavor to be added, by using ready-made spicer-uppers you can find in your supermarket.

Like the lunchtime salad, go for high quality sauces with ingredients made without chemical nonsense. Check the label to see how much of the sauce you could have on your plan, and choose some lovely sauces to add flavor to your meals.

Ideally, we'd have it all home-made. But this is the real world where time is often short, and sometimes we choose to eat something different to the rest of the family. We need it quick, convenient, tasty, and healthy.

The amount of butter and olive oil allowed simply ties in with what's been allocated for the sauce. It even surprised me, that you don't really need the measly portions allowed on some diets that unnecessarily restrict fat too much.

Having said that, don't have butter every day. It's great for the convenience and taste factor, but it is high in saturated fat. And although opinions vary on the use of butter, once every few days on the dinner meal is fine.

## WHEN YOU HIT YOUR TARGET

Ease your way back to "maintenance"—which means you can eat freely, whilst sticking to the same structure you've been using all along whilst doing the *Habit Guide* diet weight loss plans.

Say you're doing the 1250 plan. As you near your goal weight, move up to the 1500 plan for a couple of weeks, and then to the 1750 plan for a couple of weeks, before letting yourself loose and trusting your appetite to guide you from now on.

Of course, you'll be in fantastic habits by then. Nothing really changes in what you're eating. It's just all the attention to portion sizes that can stop.

## WEIGHING STUFF—A DRAG?

Not really. Cook up plenty of food at dinner time depending on what the family is doing too. Instead of dishing the food out onto your plate randomly, your plate is sitting on a kitchen scale. Is that a hassle really? Well I do it every day even though I'm not losing weight, because I do everything I ask you to do.

And it's not a hassle at all. It's easy.

Reset or "tare" the scale before each food item goes on.

Once you get the hang of the portion sizes, you can just "eyeball" your restaurant meal if you're out and about, and know you're near enough. Remember weight loss is not a sprint. It's about eating just the right amount every day consistently.

But in the house, the scale is there—why not use it? It's easy.

## WEIGH-INS

You'll need a good quality digital scale to track your progress. So beg, borrow or buy one if you haven't got one, and weigh-in once a week only.

Weight can fluctuate quite a bit for various reasons like hydration levels, monthly cycles, and so-on. So there's no need to obsess about the scale.

If you stick to the simple meal plans you're guaranteed steady weight loss. Despite folks telling me it's their genes or their thyroid that's the reason they gained weight, I've never known anything but predictable weight loss with consistent under-eating at just the right level.

If you don't lose weight on these plans you should definitely see your doctor!

Weigh-in first thing in the morning after using the bathroom and before having a drink. Put the scale out the night before if you remember, to let it settle. And wear the same type of clothing (or no clothing) each time.

## WATER LOSS

The fast weight loss in the first week or two is due to water loss. Carbohydrate is stored in your body with a lot of water. So as that carbohydrate is used for fuel, the water is released.

This is something that confuses many people. If you have a day where you're "off" the diet, you could gain a lot of weight. But don't worry, it's mainly water not fat you're gaining. It will go as quickly as it came when you get back on track.

## IF THE GOING GETS TOUGH

The plans will result in 1½ to 2 pounds a week weight loss for most people. This is the rate people want so I go along with it. But really, a better target is 1 pound a week. So, if you find you're hungry, just step to the next plan up, and you'll still lose weight.

The number one thing is *consistency,* not the rate of weight loss. I've seen study after study of clinical trials, where even with the massive support of the study, the drop-out rates and the rate of loss after a year was abysmal!

But here you have all the right solutions—habits, simplicity, consistency, structure, variety and flexibility. So, if you're struggling—please step to the next higher calorie target. Staying the course is the most important thing.

The tortoise *won* the race remember!

# six

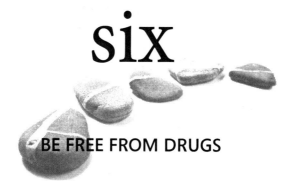

## BE FREE FROM DRUGS

*"The doctor of the future will give no medication, but will interest his patients in the care of the human frame, diet and in the cause and prevention of disease."*

—Thomas A. Edison

Although the "pill-for-an-ill" mindset still dominates today, throughout the ages, a few insightful health professionals and free-thinkers have figured out the big picture; the true causes and the true solutions to our modern diseases.

Even the "father" of modern medicine, Hippocrates, said "Let food be thy medicine." And doctors still swear the "Hippocratic Oath," but how many follow his sage advice?

We are at the beginning of a new era of widespread understanding of Hippocrates' insight so many years ago. The "lifestyle diseases" that claim most of our lives and cause so much suffering, are more and more being understood to have only a lifestyle solution.

Governments, facing massive future costs if health care doesn't change, are being forced to take action now—with campaigns to help us get the lifestyle message and change our ways.

## TRUE SOLUTIONS

In most cases if you get sick, your body is at breaking point from years, even decades of not meeting your body's needs. The solution is to meet those needs, not introduce drugs into an already out-of-balance biochemical system.

Drugs can restore a certain crude balance, but it's like adding a fog horn to a symphony orchestra.

Our aim needs to be to put the conditions in place, that allow our incredibly complex bodies to self-regulate. In the main, these conditions are the ones that existed before industry, before agriculture, before modern civilization. They are the natural conditions that were there before drugs and processed foods—fresh air, sunshine, natural food, exercise, good sleep and low stress.

## SIDE EFFECTS AND DEPENDENCY

Pharmaceutical drugs, recreational drugs and even the common drugs—caffeine and alcohol are all fog horns. All drugs have side-effects because of their crude action and some drugs cause a physiological dependency.

When you put a drug into a finely tuned system like your body, it adapts to the presence of that drug. Often a higher and higher dose is needed to get the desired effect. Or your body adapts to certain chemicals being there, and stops its own production of those chemicals.

## BIO-MAYHEM

Stopping that drug then causes biochemical mayhem until the body can re-adjust. A simple example of this is a baby who develops vitamin deficiency because her mother took high-dose supplements.

The baby's body adapted by excreting most of the vitamins and so when born, the baby still excretes high amounts of vitamins even though the supply has now stopped.

Likewise, people can become dependent on mood altering drugs—because stopping the drug makes them feel even worse than the original problem. Not only has the real cause of the problem not been addressed, but now you have a bigger problem and side effects to boot!

## ENERGY LOAN SHARK

Drugs rarely get to the root of the problem, because the problem was never lack of drugs. If you're tired, a solution is to drink a big mug of strong coffee. But caffeine is an energy loan shark. Your body knew what it was doing and what you should have done was rest.

But now you're "flogging a dead horse"—making an already tired body run at triple speed. It's amazing our bodies cope as long as they do.

And as you'll see a little later, caffeine also plays into a vicious circle that gradually steals your energy and vitality, leaving you depressed and tired all the time.

"There's no safe drug," a doctor once told me. "And all drugs have side-effects," she said.

So we need a very clear mindset. Drugs create biochemical disharmony, and should be a last resort to buy you time to sort your lifestyle out.

The whole big picture of drug use is very disturbing, involving big corporations with money, not care, as the principle driving force.

But the truth is now dawning—drugs could not, can not and will not ever solve a problem caused by poor lifestyle.

That doesn't mean you should stop taking your medicine. That could be very dangerous if unsupervised by your doctor. But if you have health conditions, you could talk to your doctor to see what the true underlying causes are—and see if there is a natural solution.

Unfortunately many doctors are not trained in, or even aware of health creation. Doctors are schooled in the art of disease, not health. The enlightened ones are self-taught. So you may need to do your own research on this, and seek out an enlightened doctor who is willing to help you work towards being drug free.

And of course, nearly everyone is "using." Too much caffeine and alcohol and other "undesirables," all place our bodies under more stress than we should be coping with.

We wouldn't do to our children what we will happily do to ourselves. Would you give strong coffee to your child? (or stress them to breaking point with late nights and overwork for that matter). I'm not a party pooper—it's the *habitual* use of common drugs that concerns me most, and the long-term suffering they cause.

I'm not against drugs per se. I'm against the use of drugs where a natural, better, cheaper and truer solution exists. I'm for solutions that actually resolve the true underlying cause of the problem.

So, for the sake of health and to feel good all the time, aim to be drug free whenever possible. And put the conditions in place that let your amazing body do the thing it's good at—keeping you happy and healthy.

# seven

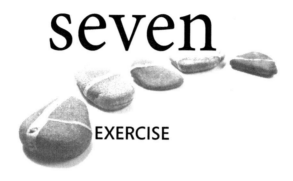

## EXERCISE

*"Better to hunt in fields, for health unbought,*
*Than fee the doctor for a nauseous draught,*
*The wise, for cure, on exercise depend;*
*God never made his work for man to mend."*

—John Dryden

## YOU'RE BUILT TO MOVE

Your genes reflect your ancestors' very active lifestyles. You're built to move, it's in your design, and if you don't exercise you'll suffer.

For example, the trillions of cells in your body are bathed in lymph, which feeds them and removes their waste. But the lymph system has no pump, unlike blood, which is pumped around by your heart. *Movement* is the pump for lymph.

Another example of how your genes reflect your design for activity is "human growth hormone" or HGH. It's the so-called "youth hormone," and it's released when you exercise. This hormone is credited with the ability to burn fat, build muscle, rejuvenate sagging skin, restore libido, and reverse memory loss!

The strength of your bones is related to how much they are "stressed." When bone is put under pressure (weight-bearing exercise) it gets stronger.

These are just three examples of how we're designed to move. There are thousands just like it. You could look at how your body works from a thousand angles and see how it adapts and changes to exercise. Science likes to cut up and dissect all these functions and effects, but when you live a natural life, everything works together naturally—a beautiful synergy.

You don't need to know how it all works. You just need to know what you need to do, and of course *how to get yourself to do it,* to get the amazing benefits of living a natural life.

## EFFORT IS NEEDED BECAUSE...

We are now separate from nature. Your ancestors didn't have to think about fitting in their exercise, or going to the gym. The pressing needs of every day forced them to do it.

So a good exercise program simply mimics the kind of movements and the intensity that your ancestors did. That will move your lymph, release HGH, build strong bones, and all the other wonderful effects. To mimic the lifestyle we're designed for at a genetic level means plenty of walking and general moving around, plus a bit of running and moving heavy stuff now and then.

Exercise advice as a whole is too complex, there's too much of it, and a lot doesn't apply to what most people want—to simply be fit and healthy—to look and feel great. And like every area of health, there's a gaping void between the amount and complexity of information out there, and what's really happening in most people's real lives.

This complexity is one of the big factors that are putting people off doing it. Another big one is that people in general, don't like doing it because it hurts too much, or they feel self-conscious. Over time, exercise can become associated in the mind with unpleasant feelings, and that just won't work in the long term. And the long term is the important time-frame.

But all these problems can be easily overcome by using habit power, controlling the intensity (how hard you're working), and by simplicity—having a simple and flexible plan that can be used for life.

Then exercise, like all the other lifestyle factors becomes an extremely enjoyable thing to do. This chapter will show you how to get the body and energy you want, without the stress and strain you may be associating with exercise.

## BENEFITS

The benefits of exercise are truly huge, but difficult to put into a few words, because there are just so many benefits and they're inter-related. To explain the benefits, they have to be categorized and the effects separated. That can be done to an extent, but it doesn't convey the synergy that's there. That, you can only imagine.

Your body functions as a whole, and every tiny part of your body benefits. Here are the big payoffs, but try to imagine that synergy—every benefit, one to another, and to all the other lifestyle elements!

- **Resistance to diseases** like heart disease, cancer, obesity, diabetes and stroke. Exercise improves circulation, strengthens your heart and lowers blood pressure and cholesterol levels.

- **More energy.**

- **Increased strength and flexibility.**

- **Better body composition** (more muscle, less fat).

- **Looking younger.** You don't only look younger, you actually *are* younger, biologically speaking—exercise can cut your biological age by up to ten years.

- **Feeling good.** Brain chemicals released during exercise, such as serotonin and endorphins, are known to have strong effects on mood. They reduce anxiety, stress and depression. A regular exercise program just makes you feel good to be in your skin!

- **Better sleep.**

- **Stronger bones.** Your bones get stronger when they are put under pressure—from "weight-bearing" exercise.

- **Detoxification** through lymph and perspiration. Your lymph system, which removes waste from your cells, relies on movement from your muscles to push the lymph around. If you don't move, your cells are sitting in their own waste!

- **Faster metabolism.** Exercise burns calories so you'll be able to eat more food without weight gain. And the extra muscle you gain also burns calories. Muscle is "metabolically active" tissue.

- **Improved immune system.**
- **Improved self-esteem.** As you look and feel better, naturally, you'll feel better about yourself.
- **Improved mental alertness** and clarity of thought.

## EXERCISE FUNDAMENTALS

YOU GET WHAT YOU TRAIN FOR

Your body is constantly adapting to your environment—amazing really. How your genes play out—which ones are switched on or off, depends on your lifestyle. Your body adapts to what you put into your mouth, as well as the physical demands you place on it. It will adapt if you work hard, and it will also adapt if you do nothing—you'll lose muscle, strength, energy, and bone strength.

So, fitness cannot be stored. You don't get to keep it. To keep fit, you have to maintain the level of activity that gives you the desired outcome for life.

The key words there are "maintain" and "life." Getting fit is a little bit harder than maintaining fitness. So, once you've achieved the level of strength, endurance, and flexibility you want... stick. Then it's easy—do it for life to get all the amazing benefits.

The way your body adapts is *very specific*. It aims to adapt, given the right resources such as nutrition and sleep, to allow you to do today, what you attempted, but struggled with yesterday.

So, to get fit, to get to that wonderful stage where all you need to do is maintain, you need to create *training effects*. What this means is attempting, briefly, something that's hard for you to do, to get your body to adapt and change. "Briefly" is the key word there because if it isn't brief, it's going to be unpleasant, and then you're back to associating exercise with unpleasant feelings again!

Remember that you only need to create training effects while you are *getting* fit. Once you *are* fit, you can stay in your comfort zone all the time.

And because we're interested in getting and staying fit for life, you only need to make small changes, small training effects. That's not unpleasant at all. By taking your time, thinking long term and managing the intensity of exercise, you get to have all the rewards easily, without the stress and strain and the "no pain-no gain."

## WARMING UP AND COOLING DOWN

Both these are essential for exercising safely. Before any exercise of even moderate intensity, your body needs to be prepared—muscles, tendons, heart, lungs and so-on. If you don't warm up properly it can lead to serious injury, and if you don't cool down properly it can lead to fainting.

## SAFE EXERCISE SEQUENCE

- Warm up 5 minutes
- Work at slightly-out-of-breath intensity for 20 minutes
- Cool down 5 minutes
- Stretch

Really, that's pretty much all there is to it. Choose an activity that can get you slightly out of breath and do it for twenty minutes.

Beginners should build up to the length of time and intensity gradually. For example, you could start with ten minutes and add five minutes every week.

If you're trying to get fit, you need to know that your workouts are effective (creating a small training effect). You can do this by monitoring the intensity—either by watching how hard you're breathing, monitoring your heart rate, or by going by how hard you feel you're working (Perceived Rate of Exertion - PRE).

Monitoring your heart rate is the most effective way to make sure that the exercise you're doing, is at the right intensity for you. It's the only method of the three that's pure information, and doesn't rely on you making a judgment.

I find that when I don't wear my heart rate monitor, I don't work as hard. It's particularly effective when doing "regular" cardio workouts such as jogging, cycling and so-on. When the competitive element of sport comes in, it's unlikely you won't work hard enough (although you may work too hard!).

Take a very unfit person and a very fit person and get them to exercise at the same level of intensity—say run together from one end of the street to the other. The unfit person's heart would be pounding out of their chest, whilst the fit person would hardly even be warmed up.

So, the heart rate monitor makes sure you're not working too hard, and not being too lazy! You're working at just the right level for you.

The heart rate monitor chest straps and watches to go with them can be bought quite cheaply.

So, now you know how to monitor your heart rate, what do you do with that information? When you're training your heart and lungs it's good to know a couple of facts and figures…

"Maximum Heart Rate" or MHR is an estimate of the fastest your heart will beat, and depends mainly on your age. There are quite a few methods around for working it out, but a simple way of estimating it that's most often used is:

MHR = 220 - age

So a 40 year old person will have an estimated maximum heart rate of 180 beats per minute (bpm).

"Target Heart Rate" or THR is the actual figure you're aiming for whilst training. Often it's written as a range of figures. The aerobic training range is usually given as 60% to 85% of MHR.

So for our 40 year old example, the range would be 60% to 85% of 180 bpm. Simply multiply your MHR by 0.6 and then 0.85 to give your aerobic training range. In our example the range is 108 to 153.

Now this is a very big range! But it's usually narrowed down depending on your fitness levels and goals. So a beginner may start off with 10 minutes at 60-65% of MHR and then go to 15 minutes at 65-70% of MHR and so-on.

If you're following the *Habit Guide* weight loss plan and you're new to exercise, then lower intensity workouts such as brisk walking may be best for you. This allows you to train for much longer, and so burn more calories.

You can train long and you can train hard, but you can't train long *and* hard.

To progress your fitness levels you can increase F.I.T.—either the Frequency, Intensity or Time (duration) of your workouts.

**Frequency**—Do more sessions.

**Intensity**—Increase the Target Heart Rate range, e.g. from 60-65% to 65-70%.

**Time**—Have longer sessions.

In practice, it's usually best to increase the intensity. Most people are not going to be able to find more time to have longer sessions, or more sessions.

As your fitness improves, your resting heart rate will be lower, due to the increased efficiency of your heart. Five-time successive Tour de France winner Miguel Indurain had a resting heart rate around 30 bpm!

Great ways to train your heart and lungs include walking (use hills to increase intensity), jogging, treadmills, cross-trainers, rowing, steps, step machines, cycling, and many sports such as soccer, badminton, tennis, and so-on.

I think intense walking (up hills) is hard to beat because walking is the most natural movement. It's low impact (doesn't jar the joints), and almost anyone can do it. Sports for me are more fun though, and I tend to work harder as I'm thinking about winning, and not how hard I'm working.

For rainy days, a simple step is my favorite, a great workout… low impact, high intensity, takes up little room and it's easy to store.

The most important thing is to work up to doing *something* for 30 minutes most days (including warm up and cool down/ stretch). Monday to Friday works well, and then you can keep your weekends free.

# eight

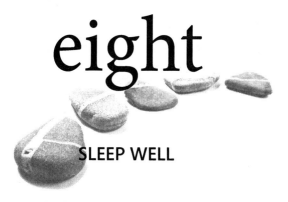

## SLEEP WELL

> "SLEEP THAT KNITS UP THE RAVELLED SLEAVE OF CARE,
> THE DEATH OF EACH DAY'S LIFE, SORE LABOUR'S BATH,
> BALM OF HURT MINDS, GREAT NATURE'S SECOND COURSE,
> CHIEF NOURISHER IN LIFE'S FEAST."

—William Shakespeare, Macbeth

Of all the lifestyle elements, perhaps none will sap your energy faster than poor quality sleep. But with the right mindset in place—making sleep a priority, and a few little tips and tricks, you can be sure of deep, restful sleep every night. This alone will make a massive difference to your health and well-being.

## A VICIOUS CIRCLE

Poor sleep, caffeine and alcohol are linked together in a vicious circle. Poor sleep leads to more stimulant use, and more stimulant use leads to poorer and poorer quality sleep. And although alcohol helps us get to sleep, our sleep quality is reduced overall.

Our biochemistry does not appreciate being tampered with by drugs, and our natural circadian rhythms are put out-of-sync by these commonly used drugs.

This vicious circle is a major cause of chronic fatigue and depression, and even if you're getting the right number of hours, this pattern—when continued over months and years, as habits tend to do, causes a tremendous loss of vitality, energy and happiness.

Once things start to spiral downward, they tend to keep going in that direction—poor sleep leading to lowered immunity, susceptibility to colds and infections, relationships strained, alcohol abuse and so-on.

So a good first step to better sleep is to reduce caffeine intake, and stay away from caffeine after 6pm at the latest. Alcohol is also best kept to small amounts; say a small glass of red wine, preferably with your evening meal.

Ideally, it's best to have no caffeine at all but if you don't want to give up your coffee or tea habit completely, 4pm is the time to have it—when it won't affect your natural circadian 24 hour cycle.

## THE RHYTHM OF SLEEP

Many people go to bed at different times each night and many dislike going to bed, and stay up way past when they should. Once the vicious circle of stimulant use and the habit of staying up late are in place, it can be surprisingly difficult to get your body to readjust.

It wasn't so long ago that our ancestors were tied to the cycles of nature. They went to bed when it went dark and got up at dawn. Our bodies thrive on these cycles because that's what they expect to happen.

So, another important step to quality sleep is to have regular times to go to bed and get up. Putting sleep as a top priority is what's going to get you to bed on time.

We can mimic the natural cycles of nature to fit in with our lives by making our rooms very dark and cool. The temperature naturally drops outside at night, so you should recreate those conditions in your bedroom. This fall in temperature is one of the signals your body uses to know it's time for sleep.

Open your bedroom window for 10 minutes as part of your normal bedtime routine, and close it before you get into bed if noise or adverse weather is likely. This way, you get to cool your room slightly, and get a good dose of fresh air in too.

Falling light levels are another signal your body uses to know it's time to sleep. So make sure you have black-out curtains or blinds in your bedroom, so street lights don't interfere with you dropping off, and early morning sunlight doesn't wake you up.

## NO WORRIES

Sleep time is not the time to think at all, much less worry. Use relaxation as part of your normal drop-off technique. After you climb into bed, imagine a huge switch and heave that lever to the OFF position. After that—no more thinking!

Take a few deep breaths, and then put all your attention into your feet. Keep your attention there for 10 or 20 seconds then move up to your calves and do the same. Gradually move up through your whole body in the same way—feeling your body from the inside, noticing tension and releasing it. If you find tension but can't release it, then squeeze that muscle tightly and release. Repeat until the tension is gone.

If you get to the top of your head and you're still awake, then start again with your feet.

It might help you at first to add an auto-suggestion… "I'm relaxing my feet, my feet are relaxed… I'm relaxing my calves…" and so-on.

After months of practicing this technique, you'll just love going into your inner body for relaxation at bedtime. It's really a wonderful experience.

## UP IN THE NIGHT

If you need to get up in the night to use the bathroom, don't put on the light, or it could upset hormonal systems in your body that start your body waking up. If there's danger of accidents without lights, then install some night lights.

## DAWN — TIME TO WAKE UP

Just as we can mimic the ideal conditions for sleep, we can wake up naturally by using a dawn simulator connected to our bedside lamp.

These hi-tech solutions are invaluable, especially if your bio-clock is very sensitive to light levels. For seasonal affective disorder (SAD) sufferers, a dawn simulator in conjunction with a light box can save months of depression.

Your bedside lamp won't be as strong as a natural dawn, but it's enough to get your body to start the process of waking up. It stops that awful feeling of the alarm going off when you're in deep sleep.

My alarm also has a groovy fade-out for bedtime where the lamp gradually dims as I'm falling asleep.

## NATURAL ALARM CLOCK

With regular sleep cycles, a dark, cool room, and a dawn simulator, pretty soon you'll be waking up about 1 minute before the alarm goes off. Quite amazing really! Instead of waking up groggy and fatigued, you'll soon be getting all the benefits of regular deep and sound sleep triggered by natural signals that you can mimic in your bedroom.

## POWER NAPS

When your healthy lifestyle is fully in place, it's very unlikely you'll need to nap during the day, but if you're coming from ill-health or trying to turn your health around, then power naps can be a powerful tool.

Keep naps to 20 minutes if possible. Although the best time to nap is between 2pm and 5pm, if you're tired, you're tired—do it whenever. A 20 minute snooze is a fantastic way to recharge your batteries and it won't affect your night-time sleep.

## SIMPLE AND POWERFUL

Good sleep is an amazing way to improve health, because it needs so little effort other than putting a few things in place and then making sure you get to bed on time.

Fantastic results for no effort, is definitely worth having. The most difficult thing is to quit the caffeine but take it a step at a time, removing the ones closest to bedtime first.

Sleep, like all the lifestyle elements, is a powerful influencer of mood. If you're looking for the best way to start your happy and healthy life changes, you could do worse than making sure you get deep, nourishing sleep, night after night. Sleep tight!

# nine

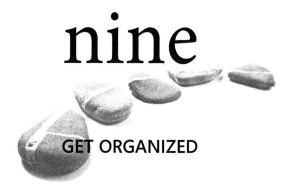

## GET ORGANIZED

*"Be careless in your dress if you will,*
*but keep a tidy soul."*

—Mark Twain

The stresses and strains on us these days are unprecedented. Is it surprising that striving for success, juggling all our things-to-do, and fire-fighting the chaos in our lives leaves us depleted?

If we want to be happy and always feel good, this situation has to change. It's essential that we take the first step and get our priorities straight. Otherwise we can waste huge amounts of energy and resources, chasing after things that cannot ever make us happy.

If your happiness depends on the idea of having or doing, then it won't make you happy in the long run, not on its own. Something fundamental will always be lacking and you'll always feel unfulfilled. The problem comes from confusing pleasure with happiness, so what's the difference?

- **Pleasure**—Temporary physical or psychological good feelings.

- **Happiness**—Contentment, appreciation, joy and love; feelings of connection to being, in this moment, now.

I know people who've spent their whole lives chasing a dream they thought would make them happy, only to achieve it and realize they were no happier than before. They put all of themselves into outer success, but their dream turned out to be an idea, a concept… "I will be happy when I have this thing" or "I will be happy when I am doing that thing."

So we chase after rainbows. How can there be lasting happiness by chasing things that come and go by their very nature?

This is about knowing clearly what can fix bad feelings and what cannot, getting to what truly matters. Putting happiness first doesn't deny pleasure, having or doing. But when you're happy for no reason, you just don't strive for pleasure, things, achievements or status as *fulfillment*.

Happy people don't stop having or doing, in fact, they often have and do with more zest. They just don't make a *self* out of it; they're not attached or needy because they're not coming from a place of lack. And so what happy people choose to have and do, are choices coming from an entirely different state of being, and a true sense of self.

## SOLID FOUNDATIONS

The first step in getting organized is to look at your dreams and desires, and really, question whether they are likely to make you happy.

By taking this first step, we can free up huge energy resources, by realizing that our happiness is not at the end of business success, a puffed up ego, or a grand house. Happiness is an inner harmonious state of health, and a deep connection to life in the present moment.

Put the horse before the cart. Get happy first, and *then* see what you do!

## DANCE IT!

Once we've got our priorities straight, it's time to systemize the day-to-day things-to-do so we can dance through it, and avoid the chaos caused by inefficiency and avoidance.

The trick is to get all the routine stuff efficiently dispatched. Imagine that dancer again—each movement practiced, effortless, each linked to the previous one in flow. We can dance through our day-to-day things-to-do like that, freeing our minds from worry about what's not been done, freeing our soul from resistance to our own lives.

## ONLY TWO TYPES OF ACTION

Everything you do is either a *regular action* that needs doing every day or every week, or it's a *one-off action*. So we can free our minds by creating two lists—"regular actions" and "one-off actions."

## REGULAR ACTIONS

This is your daily and weekly routine that efficiently dispatches the stuff to keep your life running smoothly, and allows you to forget the boring stuff—safe in the knowledge that everything is taken care of.

Your regular actions list is always a work-in-progress. As your life changes or your aims change, you simply tweak your regular actions list to reflect the new conditions.

It's what you do from morning to night. Regular actions listed in an order meaningful to you, that you simply dance your way through.

On that list is everything that needs to be done to maintain the status quo, and move you forward into the vision of what you're trying to create for your life. Woody Allen famously said "99% of success is showing up." In your regular actions you "show up" consistently for those things that need your regular attention.

See how much you relax when it's all taken care of consistently. Washing is done, kids are fed, fridge is stocked, house is clean and car is serviced. Then we can forget about all that boring stuff and get on with living.

### GETTING STARTED

Draw up a list—be the choreographer of your dance. What do you want your day to look like from morning to night? Then, start to put it into action—dance it. Go through the list, one thing after another, each activity *linked* to the next in a smooth, efficient flow.

### IT'S GREAT WHEN BAD THINGS HAPPEN

When bad things happen, it's generally because we weren't proactive—we didn't take action soon enough to prevent disaster. For example; you get home from work tired and hungry, the kids are screaming for food, and there's nothing in the fridge. When bad stuff happens, it's a great opportunity to think "What needed to be on my regular actions list that would have prevented this?"

As time goes by, all those chaotic annoyances that cause us unnecessary stress simply disappear. This isn't about being too controlling, it's about doing what needs to be done, as efficiently as possible.

## ONE-OFF ACTIONS

After you've finished dancing your way through your regular actions, it's time to look at the "one-offs."

All your projects and one-off things-to-do can go here in nested lists, that boil down the outcomes you want into very precise, doable actions.

For example;

**Sell house**

> Contact agent

>> Which one?

>>> Talk to Jessie about that

**Finish re-tiling the bathroom**

> Buy more grout

Once you've narrowed each outcome down into the smallest doable actions, you can copy the "next actions today" onto another piece of paper. Here, the next actions today are to talk to Jessie about which agent to use, and buy some grout.

## BANG, BANG, BANG

These two lists will supercharge your doing power and free your mind from worry. It's wonderful to get it all into a system because to be happy here and now, we need to feel safe, that all is OK, it's all taken care of. How can we laugh and enjoy life if we're burdened by worry and concern?

Boil everything down into doable actions. If you find yourself worrying—stop! Ask yourself "What can I actually *do* about this?" "What is the outcome I want in this situation?"

Your answers to those questions can be put on either the regular actions or one-off actions lists, and instead of worrying, you can take efficient action or let it go.

# ten

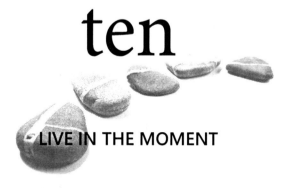

## LIVE IN THE MOMENT

*"Let anyone try, I will not say to arrest, but to notice or to attend to, the present moment of time. One of the most baffling experiences occurs. Where is it, this present? It has melted in our grasp, fled ere we could touch it, gone in the instant of becoming."*

—William James

We're living half-lives at best if we give most of our attention to the abstract world of thought, and miss life itself—which is only found in the present moment.

Learning to re-connect to the present moment is one of the most essential disciplines to allow happiness to happen. It's actually incredibly difficult to do because we are *habitually* thinking. It's become second nature. As soon as our eyes open in the morning, the constant stream of thinking starts and doesn't stop until we go into deep sleep again.

Imagine you're 5 years old again, on the beach playing with a stick making shapes in the sand. How happy you are! And where is your attention? What is your experience? Are there any thoughts, worries, roles or status?

Is there a "me" in there that isn't just your very being? Isn't everything just happening? Isn't life just flowing? Aren't you really just aware of yourself playing? How strange!

As children, our experience is whole—mind, body and spirit in flow. We were flow-ers, delightful—full of light. That's the quality that all spiritual traditions try to describe, and the quality they try to achieve. But can "light" be described? Can love be described? They can only be *experienced.*

We must reconnect to that light, to the indescribable depth of our being—the love that we are in essence. We must learn to stop our attention being dragged into the abstract world of thinking without our say so—thinking that makes us slaves and creates the illusion of ego, like dense clouds that cover up the sun.

It's actually very simple—we need to stop the mind-chatter. When the mind-chatter stops, you're in the present moment. But it's also very difficult to do, so we need some solid techniques to practice, to relearn how to be present for our life.

Thinking needs to be relegated back to its proper place as a *doing.* It's a doing, like walking. You know how to stop walking but can you stop thinking? If not, then you're a slave to thinking, not the master.

Thoughts are creative movements of energy, they have a lot of power. We are moving into the vision created by our thinking, so we need to be the master of that. If we're thinking haphazardly, then our lives will reflect that chaotic inner state.

To put thinking back into its proper place as a choiceful activity is a beautiful thing. Then happiness is what's left—freedom, spontaneity and the joy of simply being. Because at the deepest level that being-ness is love itself.

The more your attention can rest in the *essence* of who you really are, the happier you will be, the more de-lighted and the more love and compassion will flow through you, into your life.

## STOPPING THE MIND-CHATTER

First we relearn to get back to "no-mind," then we can relearn how to flow. There are lots of ways to get the mind to shut up. The one I favor is simply to *listen*.

Normal thinking is similar to a song playing in our heads that we can't stop. But as soon as you become alert and listen, you interrupt the whole process. Play musical statues with your own mind. Listen intensely for the next thought (the music to start playing again) and an amazing thing happens; the thoughts stop!

Listening is actually a higher state of consciousness. Normal thinking is only a semi-conscious activity. It sucks in all our attention and we get dragged along. And the amazing irony is that we believe all this thinking is actually *us*.

This identification with thinking is our ego—a very destructive false sense of self that does nothing but damage in our lives.

But if you stop the mind-chatter, the ego disappears because the ego is the illusion of a million thoughts we incorrectly called "me."

## LISTENING IS SIMPLY BEING

Tune in to the real you—the "you" obscured by incessant mental noise. It's a very simple technique—you listen intently enough to "catch" the next thought that comes. It's this process of stepping back and listening, that stops all your attention being sucked into thinking itself.

When you're relaxed, alert and centered—when your attention is on the *space* in which thought happens—thoughts come up naturally at just the right time that you need them.

When you practice the art of listening, what feels strange at first becomes a joy—an infinitely better way of being and living. It's a beautiful simplicity that makes everything shiny and new again.

## INTENSE PRACTICE—MEDITATION

In our normal lives, we have a lot of "input" coming at us all day—sights, sounds, deadlines, this, that, the other. All this makes stopping the mind-chatter harder, because all this input is triggering thoughts.

So it's great to find some quiet time to learn the art of listening—tuning into the space in which thought happens.

Whenever you get the opportunity for a few quiet minutes, close your eyes and take a few deep breaths. Move your attention into your body and feel and release any tension there. Let thoughts come and go without following, without judgment. And let everything settle down until all there is left is pure, simple awareness.

When you get the hang of this, you'll be able to put thinking back into its proper place as a "doing," and so bring more light, more happiness and more life into the here and now.

## FLOW

Once you're able to still your thoughts, you can begin to practice paying full attention to what you're doing right here and now. And then everything becomes a meditation. It's simply holding the awareness of what you're doing.

To start, pick certain tasks to really focus on, and practice the art of flow—washing the dishes, walking up the stairs and so-on. Because we're wired for habits, you'll be reminded of your intention every time you come to do these activities.

As time goes by, add more and more activities where you focus on your flow, and in this way, your whole life will become joyful. Even tasks considered mundane such as mopping the floor will be joyful. You'll become spontaneous as your attention is totally now, and you flow from the fullness of who you are. The depth of your experience depends on how quiet your inner world is. The more still your mind, the more fully you experience life.

So, go in before flowing out. Keep listening to get back to no-mind at will. Then pay full attention to your doing, your flow. Make everything a meditation.

## HOW TO THINK

At first, getting to no-mind feels like holding back the tide but sure enough, it becomes natural and effortless and who you naturally are, is able to flow. From this place, thinking can become a conscious and deliberate doing. And as thinking is creative, that is a very good thing! It's fine and enjoyable to think and create, but be sure to do it consciously and deliberately.

Attention is how you choose, so be very careful where you put it! In your mind a thing is either there, or it isn't, so be sure your thoughts are purely about what you're trying to create and not about things you don't want. If you carry on paying attention to unwanted things, you're activating negativity in your here and now. Either think nothing, or think about things you love or want to create.

When thinking about wanted things, be sure there's no craving, hankering, or dissatisfaction, as again, you will be activating these feelings here and now. Your vision is simply an imagining of the end-state, and so will always feel only good to you.

No-mind, flow and choiceful thinking. These incredible tools remove the obstacles to a joyful and happy life.

# eleven

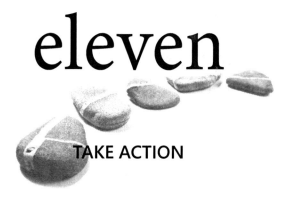

## TAKE ACTION

*"THE VISION MUST BE FOLLOWED BY THE VENTURE.*
*IT IS NOT ENOUGH TO STARE UP THE STEPS—WE*
*MUST STEP UP THE STAIRS."*

—Vance Havner

Creating health and happiness is about committing to a series of steps that put the conditions for happiness in place—the six lifestyle elements.

Although we want it all now, big steps rarely work, so take manageable steps and make each week count. Take steps you can follow through with, and make them into pacts—clear and calm decisions.

To begin, create your lifestyle blueprint—decide what you want the finish line to be for each lifestyle element, and figure out your next step for each. Pick one or two steps, make them into pacts and begin—make your start.

Here's a great affirmation to remember…

## "The most important thing I can do today is stick to my pact!"

It's the most important thing because it's staying faithful to your steps, your decisions, your pacts, that will increase your self-belief, and move you tenaciously to your finish line.

Write down each pact with the date you started underneath your lifestyle blueprint, as a record of your journey to health and happiness.

A good place to start is to get one or two weeks of enough quality sleep. It's a nightmare dragging around trying to do healthy things otherwise.

As well as good sleep habits as a fantastic first step, it's a great idea to make a start on your regular and one-off actions lists, which will rapidly remove chaos and worry from your life. Any steps you take that involve creating new good habits, or setting things up (e.g. buying things you need) can be put on your regular and one-off actions lists.

Living in the moment can also be started right away. As strange as it may seem, you don't need to think in order to act. Awareness holds thinking, not the other way around. So insist on a quiet mind, and any thinking you want to do can be done from there—consciously and deliberately.

When each lifestyle element is a mastered good habit, and is bedded into your life, you'll be happy. It cannot be any other way. You cannot be healthy, and live in the moment, and feel anything other than joy for life. This can be your constant state.

But it takes faith.

Faith is the belief in things yet unseen. Sometimes we have no frame of reference, and have been suffering for so long that we've forgotten the innocent joy of health and happiness that children have. Sometimes we need to push through minor discomforts and carefully manage our steps, even though we don't immediately get the rewards of our efforts.

So as you push through any discomforts and find your way back to happiness, keep faith in your heart—that when all these things are practiced and bedded in as good habits, and when your bad habits are a distant memory, you'll be happy.

A happy and healthy lifestyle can be hard to achieve, but it's *easy* to keep.

You deserve to be happy. Keep the faith.

## DANCE THROUGH YOUR LIST AND KEEP YOUR MIND OFF THE PINK ELEPHANT

Wherever you are on your journey, you'll want to be dancing through your regular and one-off actions, with your current steps, and everything else that needs your attention broken down into doable actions.

And keep your mind off the pink elephant—those bad habits you want to stop. Remember, you can't tell your mind not to think about something, so deal with bad habits *only* when they pop up and drop "the problem"—having faith that your sure-footed steps will take you to your desired finish line.

If your pink elephant shows up, *ignore* it—have a "don't care" attitude, and bring your mind back to what you were doing as quickly as possible. As long as you haven't picked a step that's too big, this will work like a charm. Your confidence will quickly sky-rocket, as you begin to believe in your ability to change and direct your life.

## THE ALCHEMY OF HAPPINESS

The six lifestyle elements bound together by the subtle power of habit, are the powerful causes of happiness. Instead of stress and struggle, life becomes a joy. When the lifestyle elements are effortlessly in place every day, you'll be getting all the amazing benefits—you'll be healthy, energetic, clear and free from worry. Happy!

# THANK YOU

Thank you for reading and following *Habit Guide*. I've really enjoyed bringing it to you, and I hope you've enjoyed reading it just as much.

I wish you great success with your lifestyle changes. If you're new to health, I think you'll be amazed at just how good you can feel, when you give your body and soul what they need every day.

A fantastic habit to get into, is to read a little bit of *Habit Guide* every day. This regular attention will clarify your vision and give you a regular boost of inspiration. It will also solidify your intention to get rid of the bad habits, and create the good habits that lead to health and happiness, to always *feeling good*.

Another great way to get all these benefits, is to receive our free *Habit Guide Insights* by email, which is a little nugget from *Habit Guide* each week—quick reminders to help keep you focused and on track with what works. You can sign up for them here…

www.habitguide.com/insights

And if you have any questions or feedback about *Habit Guide*, then please feel free to contact me via our website…

www.habitguide.com/contact-us

I wish you happiness always.

Good luck!

Lightning Source UK Ltd.
Milton Keynes UK
UKOW022120291211

184469UK00004B/6/P